T0284225

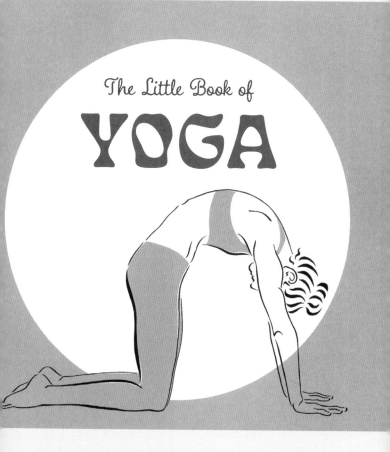

The Little Book of

YOGA

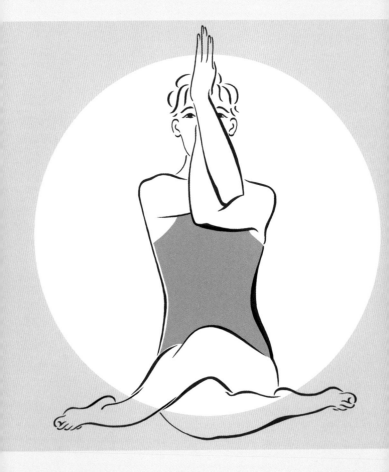

The Little Book of

YOGA

Revitalize your body, mind, and spirit

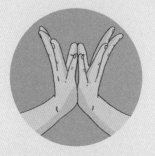

Christine Burke

CICO BOOKS
LONDON NEW YORK

Published in 2025 by CICO Books
An imprint of Ryland Peters & Small Ltd

20–21 Jockey's Fields   1452 Davis Bugg Road
London WC1R 4BW   Warrenton, NC 27589

www.rylandpeters.com

10 9 8 7 6 5 4 3 2 1

Text in this book originally featured in *The Yoga Healer*
and *The Power of Breath and Hand Yoga*

A CIP catalog record for this book is available from the
Library of Congress and the British Library.

ISBN: 978-1-80065-400-6

Printed in China

Important health note

Please be aware that the information contained in this book and the
opinions of the author are not a substitute for medical attention from
a qualified health professional. If you are suffering from any medical
complaint or are worried about any aspect of your health, or if you
are pregnant, please ask your doctor's advice before proceeding.
The publisher and author can take no responsibility for any injury or
illness resulting from the advice given or the techniques or postures
demonstrated within this volume.

Illustrators: Cathy Brear, Dionne Kitching, and Robyn Mclennan
Assistant editor: Danielle Rawlings
Commissioning editor: Kristine Pidkameny
Design concept: Maeve Bargman
Senior designer: Emily Breen
Art director: Sally Powell
Production manager: Gordana Simakovic
Publishing manager: Carmel Edmonds

MIX
Paper | Supporting
responsible forestry
FSC® C106563

contents

introduction 6

introduction

"Sthira Sukham Asanam—Steady, stable, happiness, ease in the posture"

From the Yoga Sutras of Patanjali

Yoga is OLD—very old, roughly 6,000 years old—yet it is gaining popularity faster than you can say Namaste. This is because the themes and the practice of yoga are universal and timeless. Despite all the changes that have taken place over the centuries, whether magnificent or frightening, humanity has remained fundamentally the same. We long for connection and love, health and prosperity, peace and joy.

Yoga has a long list of benefits both physical and psychological. A yoga practice can improve posture, strengthen muscles, increase flexibility, lower blood pressure, decrease the likelihood of injury, improve lung capacity, relieve anxiety, lower stress levels, increase energy levels, and enhance mental clarity. The list goes on! Not only that, but simply working with your breath and hands can be portals to self-discovery, healing, and inner peace, as you stimulate the flow of prana (life force or energy) throughout the body.

We all have difficult moments, experience stress and loss, suffer temporary or chronic physical pain, and struggle with less than graceful moods at times. Wouldn't it be wonderful to carry around a tool belt filled with everything you need to address the various conditions that arise in the course of a regular day? With yoga, you do. Scientific studies have shown that practicing certain poses (asanas), breath practices (pranayama), certain gestures and seals (mudras), and meditation to quieten the chatter of the mind results in significant benefits for the body, mind, and spirit. You can literally practice a breathing technique or short series of poses and get moving in the direction of feeling better right away—and I will show you how in this book.

The yoga in this book is hatha yoga as I practice and teach it. It is a simmering stew of all things yoga, based in tradition, and prepared for you with experience, love, humor, and passion. I have been blessed to share yoga with thousands of students and I have been fortunate to witness transformation and evolution every day. Whether you are a newcomer to yoga or a seasoned yogi, my prayer is that you will become more deeply acquainted with the healer in you, and that this relationship will infuse your life with wellbeing and many days of being well.

terminology

I have provided the English and Sanskrit names for poses, mudras, and breath practices where they first appear—while many are referred to by their English name, there are some where the Sanskrit name is used more regularly in yoga classes.

GETTING STARTED

While a traditional practice of one- or two-hour sessions is certainly something to consider and incorporate into your schedule if you can, there is much to be gained from brevity and consistency as well. Never underestimate how the power of a few focused minutes can transform your health and your outlook.

EQUIPMENT YOU WILL NEED

One of the best things about yoga is that it can be practiced anywhere and in any way. That being said, some things that will make it easier and more comfortable are:

- a yoga mat

- a yoga blanket and/or bolster

- two yoga blocks

- a yoga strap

Wear comfortable clothing, without zippers or buttons, that you would normally wear to exercise in.

You can find what you need online or in your local yoga studio. Some health food stores often sell yoga equipment, too. Feel free to get creative, and never let a lack of props stand in your way of practicing yoga. If you can breathe, you can practice.

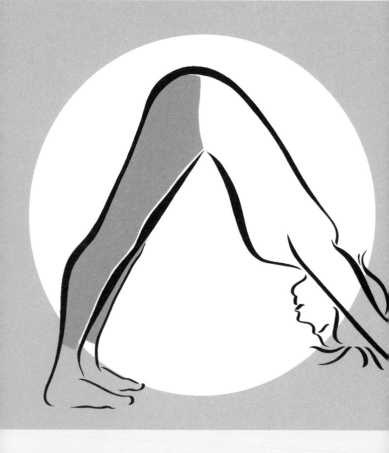

chapter one

key yoga poses

This section describes foundational poses that will come up frequently in the book. It's a good idea to familiarize yourself with them. Take your time, relax, and let them unfold for you over time— they are not something to be conquered but something to be experienced.

dandasana
(staff pose)

This may look like simply like a way of sitting down on the floor, but as with all yoga poses, it's important to take care with your position and posture to feel the full benefits.

- Sit with your legs together straight out in front of you, and with your feet flexed (toes pointing to the sky). Sit toward the front of your sitting bones so that you don't slump into your lower back.

- Place your hands alongside your hips on the floor. Your arms may be bent or straight with your palms or fingertips on the floor.

- Keep your spine straight and press your legs down toward the ground.

If you feel lower back strain, you may find it more comfortable sitting on a folded blanket.

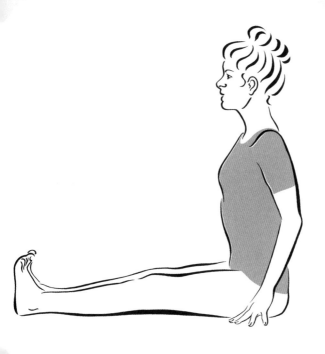

tadasana
(mountain pose)

This pose is about standing with intention, firm as a mountain.

- Stand up tall with your feet together and your arms extending energetically by your sides.

- Balance on each foot equally from the inner to the outer, from the ball to the heel.

- Firm your legs.

- Set a focus point (*Drishti*) in the near distance in front of you at eye height.

- Keep the chest open, the shoulders back and down.

focus/gazing point (drishti)

Set your eyes on one point in order to improve concentration and balance, and cultivate peace of mind.

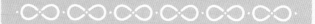

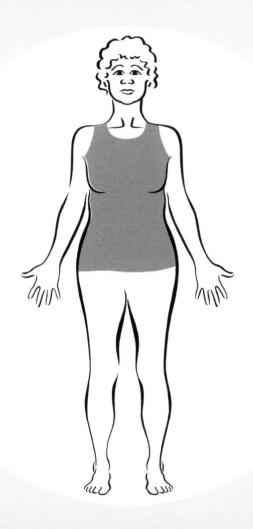

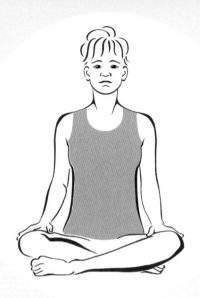

sukhasana

(easy pose)

This simple pose aids in opening the hips and aligning the spine, and its simplicity makes it suitable for yogis of all skill levels.

- Sit with your legs straight out in front of you in *Dandasana* (see page 12).

- Bend one leg and bring it in.

- Bend the other leg and cross it over the first one. Your legs should be crossed at the shins, and when you look down you should see a triangle between your legs.

- Keep a comfortable gap between your feet and your pelvis.

You may wish to sit up on a folded blanket to avoid compression in the lower back, or tuck a blanket under your knees for more support.

ALTERNATIVE POSE:

siddhasana (accomplished pose)

This pose is a bit more advanced. Begin in the same way as for *Sukhasana*, but when you bend your first leg, bring in the foot so that it lies snug to the opposite thigh. When you bend the other leg, the foot tucks in between the opposite calf and thigh. It's as if you are hiding your feet.

Another option is a loose *Siddhasana*, where the legs are open wider than in *Sukhasana* and the feet are not tucked in but on the floor in front of you with the heels lining up.

tabletop pose
(bitilasana)

This pose helps bring balance to your body and stretch all of your muscles equally.

• Simply come to all fours, placing hands under shoulders with fingers spread wide and knees under hips with the tops of the feet on the floor.

Although the closest translation in Sanskrit is *Bitilasana*, Cow Pose (see page 86), in this version the back is flat, not arched.

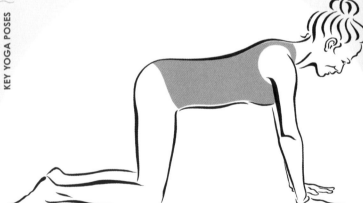

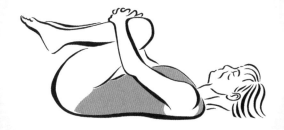

hugging knees to chest

(apanasana)

This pose is a wonderful way to release the low back.

- Lie on your back and draw your knees in toward your chest.

- Wrap your arms around your legs and hug them as close as is comfortable for your knees.

- Keep your shoulder blades and head on the floor.

standing forward fold

(uttanasana)

With this deep and satisfying stretch, it's more important to gently stretch your muscles than touch your toes.

- Stand in *Tadasana* (see page 14) with your feet either together or hip-width apart, and place your hands on your hips.

- Breathe in and as you exhale, fold forward toward the floor, bending at the hips and aligning them over your ankles. Bend your knees if your back is sensitive or your hamstrings feel too tight.

- Release your hands and clasp your elbows or place your hands either on your thighs or on the floor near the outer edges of your feet.

- Keep your legs engaged and the shoulder blades pressed firmly into your back and moving away from your ears.

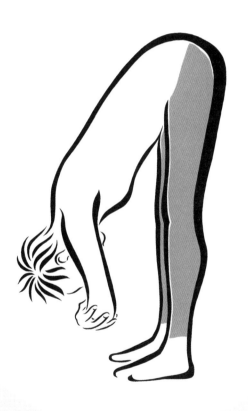

downward dog
(adho mukha svanasana)

In this pose, focus more on keeping your spine straight than your legs.

- Begin on hands and knees in Tabletop Pose (see page 18) with your hands directly under your shoulders, fingers spread wide like starfish, and your knees placed directly under your hips.

- Soften the space between your shoulder blades (think of a hammock) and engage your belly button. Without moving your hands, squeeze the arms toward each other and you will feel your biceps and triceps wake up.

- On an inhale, raise your hips and begin to straighten your legs. Push your chest toward your thighs and your heels toward the floor.

- Rotate your inner elbows to face toward each other. If you have very flexible or even double-jointed elbow joints, bend your elbows out slightly until the arms appear straight to the eye. This will engage the arms and protect the joints.

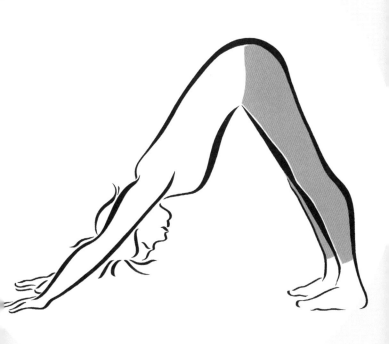

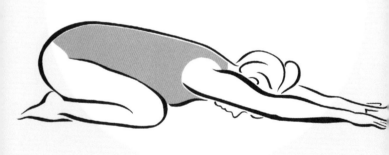

child's pose
(adho mukha virasana)

This pose stretches your neck, lower back, thighs, and ankles, while also releasing your hips.

- Start on hands and knees and bring your big toes together, shifting your knees apart so that they are wider than your hips.

- On an exhale, draw your navel toward your spine, creating a dome in your back, as you ease your hips onto your heels. This creates more space in the lower back.

- Once you are settled, allow your back to flatten out naturally as you nestle into the pose. Your forehead is on the floor with your chin tucked in and the back of the neck long. You can leave your arms stretched out in front of you, hands flat on the floor and fingers spread wide like starfish, or lay them alongside your legs with your hands near your heels, palms up.

- If your hips are high or you have trouble reaching the floor with your head, use a support, such as a folded blanket or block, under your forehead.

- If this pose is uncomfortable for your knees, you can use a bolster or folded blanket as a support: pull it into your pelvis and lay your torso along the support with your head turned to one side; your arms can be alongside your body with the palms facing up, or bring them forward, bend the elbows and "hug" the bolster.

- If your knees are still uncomfortable, roll up a blanket, towel, or article of clothing and place it snugly behind both knees before lowering your hips.

ALTERNATIVE POSE: **balasana**

Begin on hands and knees, but keep your legs together as you draw the navel to the spine and ease your hips onto your feet. As with Child's Pose, you can leave the arms outstretched or lay them alongside your legs, palms facing up.

supine twist
(supta matsyendrasana)

This pose translates as Reclining Lord of the Fishes and is great for releasing muscular tension in the upper and middle back.

- Lie on your back with your knees drawn into your chest.

- Keep your left hand on your right knee and stretch your right arm out to the right at shoulder height.

- Shift your hips slightly to the right and, as you exhale, draw your right knee across your body to the left.

- Turn your head to the right. Keep your shoulder blades in contact with the floor and your chest open and facing upward.

- Repeat on the other side.

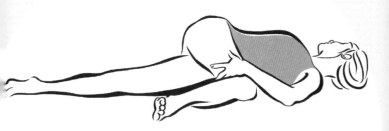

savasana

(corpse pose)

This may look like you're simply lying on the floor, but it's designed to properly let your body rest as you focus on your breathing and wind down after yoga practice.

- Lie on your back with your head in line with your spine.

- Spread your legs apart, a little wider than your hips, with your feet rolling slightly open in a natural position.

- Extend your arms away from your body (about 8 inches/20 centimeters) with the palms facing up.

- Close your eyes and breathe naturally. Relax.

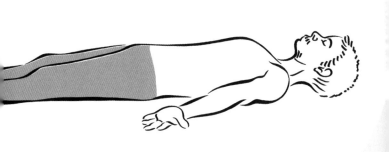

warm-up sequence

Here is a sequence that you can use to warm up before any of the remedies in the book.

SUN SALUTATIONS B VARIATION
(SURYA NAMASKAR)

1. Stand in *Tadasana* (see page 14) with your feet together or hip-width apart, and bring your hands together in prayer position over your heart center (this is *Anjali Mudra*).

2. On an inhale, sweep the arms out to the sides and overhead. As you exhale, bend forward from the hips into Standing Forward Fold (see page 20). Bend your knees if your back is tender.

3. Inhale and lift up your chest, lengthening your spine. Your arms are straight, and your hands are touching either the floor or your shins. This is a Standing Half Forward Fold.

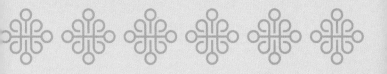

4. Exhale and fold forward again into a Standing Forward Fold.

5. Inhale to lift up your arms and bend at the hips, knees, and ankles, lowering your rear while stretching the torso upward. Exhale. Keep your arms active and in line with your ears—don't let them drift forward. This is Chair or Powerful Pose (see page 98). Hold for 1–3 breaths.

6. On your next inhale, lift straight up to standing, pushing firmly into your feet, arms stretching to the sky. Exhale as you bring your hands back to prayer position over your heart center.

7. Let your breath guide you into a rhythm and repeat this sequence as many times as you like with a minimum of 5 cycles.

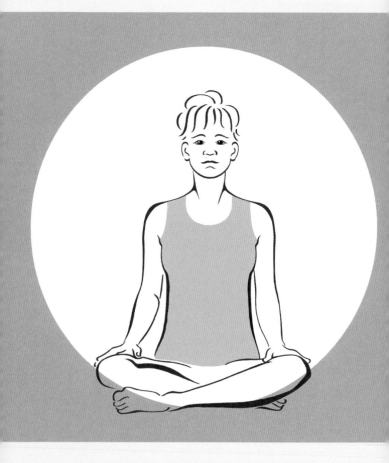

chapter two

breathing techniques

In this section, you will find a way to become aware of your breath plus breath techniques to practice. When we feel and connect with the breath, we become conscious of the rhythm of life.

breath is life

The breath is like the sky, so omnipresent that we almost forget it's there. However, when we turn our inner gaze upon our breathing and begin to notice it, feel it, hear it, and enjoy it, we experience life in a different way.

On a physical level, yogic science says that we can improve the functioning of the body by cleansing the 72,000 energy channels (nadis) and 7 energy centers (chakras, see page 142). The channels of energy move our life force (prana) and when they are cleansed, they stay fluid and clear like a fresh, beautifully running river. When we practice pranayama (see opposite page), we are enriching our blood with more oxygen, which purifies the blood and supports the healthy functioning of the respiratory system, as well as fueling the burning of glucose. These actions produce energy, which gives power to the muscular contractions of the body.

If we want to climb a mountain, we must consider our breathing capacity and our body must respond efficiently to give us the energy and strength required. If we want to relax, we can turn to the breath as well. It is a centerpiece to all that we are and all that we do and is connected to every aspect of human experience, yet we often don't think of it at all.

We live in a wonderful age of expansion and understanding where it is becoming widely recognized by traditional, functional, and alternative medical practitioners and healing specialists that breath practice can reduce anxiety and depression, lower stress levels, balance blood pressure, increase energy levels, improve sleep, and aid in pain management, among other benefits. Over the course of 31 years, it has been my personal experience and observation that all of this and more is true—each breath is a precious gift.

PRANAYAMA

Prana (life force) yama (restrain or control) is the practice of controlling the breath through various techniques toward a particular goal, such as relaxation or energizing or balancing the body, mind, and spirit. Prana is translated as life force, vitality, and essence. It can be thought of as that which animates our being, and the breath is the way we finesse and fine-tune our life force. There are many more pranayama techniques than those offered in this book, but these are the ones I come back to time and again in my teaching and personal practice, and I find them to be essential.

how to breathe

"Huh? Wait, don't I already know? I'm alive!" Yes, this is true and you have done a fine job so far. Now we will take it to the next level with pranayama and go from survival to thrival! We take the gift of our own breath and direct it for our own purpose, be that to wake up, slow down, focus, or something else.

WHAT TO DO WITH YOUR BODY WHILE YOU BREATHE

While you can breathe in any position as we do every day throughout our life, there are optimum positions for focused breath techniques. Whatever position you choose, it is most important that you are comfortable and relaxed.

SITTING

This can be in a chair or on the floor. If you are in a chair, make sure you have both feet on the ground and you are sitting upright and balanced.

If you are on the floor, you can sit in cross-legged *Sukhasana* (see page 16), either flat on the ground or on a bolster or folded blanket so you are slightly elevated. If your hips or knees feel uncomfortable, I suggest a yoga block or rolled towels, blankets, or pillows, evenly placed under each outer knee.

Another seated position is Thunderbolt Pose (see page 128). In this pose you rest on the shins with the tops of the feet on the floor and buttocks on heels. Your legs are together and your spine is straight. This pose stretches the legs and ankles and strengthens your spine. If your knees are uncomfortable, choose another position.

STANDING

If practicing while standing, have both feet evenly placed on the ground, hip-width apart if possible, stomach slightly drawn in, tailbone descending, and spine tall and straight. This is a modified *Tadasana* (see page 14).

LYING DOWN

Lying down is fine for some simple breath techniques but it is not the best position for many of them because the main energy channel for the body (*Sushumna Nadi*) is best accessed when the spine is upright and straight. However, in a few cases I suggest you rest on the floor in *Savasana* (see page 28). Your whole body is in a relaxed state, free of muscular tension.

breath practices

Get ready for a pranayama buffet! As with all aspects of yoga, it is important to approach your breathing practice free from tension. The breath affects and influences every cell in the body so a compassionate and patient approach is key for maximum benefits.

ABCS OF BREATH PRACTICE

For timing, I refer mostly to "rounds" of breath and on occasion to number of minutes. A round is one inhale and one exhale. If practicing the breath on its own, a general rule of thumb is to start with 10–30 rounds, which will take around 1–3 minutes.

You may close your eyes during the breath work or keep them open with a soft gaze fixed on one particular spot (*Drishti*, see page 14).

Unless otherwise stated for certain breath practices, breathe in and out through your nose.

breath awareness

Become aware of your breath and holding that attention on purpose.

- Gently but firmly direct your attention, as many times as it takes, with patience, toward your breath.

- Feel the sensation of the breath in your body, wherever you notice it, as it comes and goes through your nose. You may find it helpful to direct your focus to a specific area, such as your belly or chest or nostrils.

- You do not need to alter your breath but simply observe your natural breathing and passively allow your thoughts to move along without attaching to any particular thought for any length of time. Instead, attach your mind to your breath. This is a perfect way to begin to meditate.

simple equal breath

(sama vritti pranayama)

Aside from Breath Awareness (see page 39), this simplified version of Equal Breath is the easiest of the breath techniques and is an excellent choice for stress reduction. It is a perfect breath for children and teens as well.

- After a few moments of Breath Awareness, begin to count to four in your mind as you inhale through your nose.

- Pause briefly and count to four silently as you exhale through your nose.

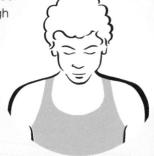

1..2..3..4

ujjayi pranayama
(triumphant/victorious breath)

This breath practice builds upon Breath Awareness (see page 39) but adds sound and action to hold your attention more firmly to the breath and therefore the present moment. In this way, you "triumph" over the chatter of the mind. It is the most common breath used in a yoga class to help you to deepen your concentration and to achieve a greater mind-body connection. This can facilitate more depth, progress, and healing in the postures.

- On your inhale "hug" or slightly constrict your throat so that it sounds like wind in a tunnel or "whoosh" and on your exhale, push the breath out through the same "hug" in the back of your throat. It should feel as if you are breathing in and out of a nose in your throat rather than your nostrils. These breaths are longer and deeper than your natural breath.

- You may also combine *Ujjayi* Breath with Equal Breath by adding the count of four. This is especially helpful for those extra busy mind moments.

three-part breath
(dirga pranayama)

The Three-part Breath is stress relieving and grounding.

- For this practice visualization is helpful. Imagine filling a glass of water from bottom to top as you fill yourself with breath.

- Inhale into the bottom of the belly, then your solar plexus (see page 143), finishing the breath in your chest.

- Pause briefly when you have filled your glass.

- Exhale from the upper chest, solar plexus, and finally bottom of the belly as if you were pouring the water from the glass.

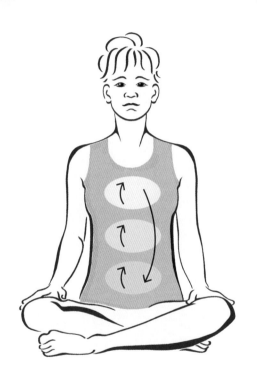

sun breath
(surya bhedana pranayama)

With this breathing technique, which is sometimes called Right Nostril Breathing, we invoke the energy of the sun. This breath can cultivate perseverance, enthusiasm, and zeal, and renew your hope.

- From a seated position, place your left hand on your thigh.

- Fold the index and middle finger of your right hand into your palm leaving the thumb, ring finger, and pinky fingers free (this is *Vishnu Mudra*). You can do this with your left hand if you are left-handed.

- Close your left nostril with your ring finger and inhale through the right nostril. Then gently pinch both nostrils shut, using the thumb on the right nostril, and pause for a few seconds with both nostrils closed.

- Lift the ring finger from the left nostril and exhale through it.

- Continue so that you always inhale through the right and exhale through the left.

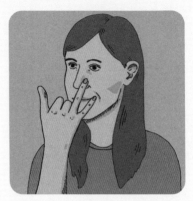

Inhale...

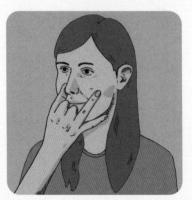

Exhale...

moon breath
(chandra bhedana pranayama)

This breathing technique, which is sometimes called Left Nostril Breathing, is cooling to the body and mind.

- From a seated position, place your left hand on your thigh.

- Fold the index and middle finger of your right hand into your palm leaving the thumb, ring finger, and pinky fingers free (this is *Vishnu Mudra*). You can do this with your left hand if you are left-handed.

- Close your right nostril with your thumb and inhale through the left nostril. Then gently pinch both nostrils shut, using the ring finger on the left nostril, and pause for a few seconds with both nostrils closed.

- Lift the thumb from the right nostril and exhale through it.

- Continue so that you always inhale through the left and exhale through the right.

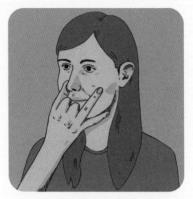

Inhale...

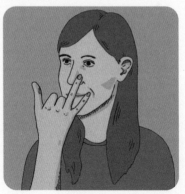

Exhale...

alternate nostril breath
(nadi shodhana pranayama)

This pranayama technique clears the two main energy channels of the body and balances the hemispheres of the brain, which can result in greater energy and focus. It is sometimes called Sun/Moon Breath.

- Sit comfortably and position your left hand, facing up or down on your leg (if you prefer a mudra, touch the thumb to the index finger in *Jnana* or *Chin Mudra*—*Jnana* is facing up, *Chin* is facing down).

- As with Sun Breath (see page 44) and Moon Breath (see page 46), take *Vishnu Mudra*: fold the index and middle finger of your right hand into your palm leaving the thumb, ring finger, and pinky finger free.

- Close your right nostril with your thumb, and inhale deeply through your left nostril. At the top of your inhale place the ring finger of your right hand over your left nostril, gently pinching the nose and pausing the breath.

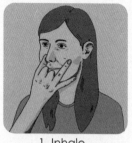
1. Inhale...

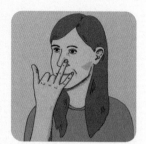
2. Exhale...

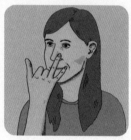
3. Inhale...

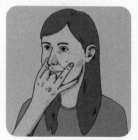
4. Exhale...

- Release your thumb and exhale through the right nostril.

- Inhale through the right nostril, close both, and exhale through the left. This is one cycle or round.

bellows breath
(bhastrika pranayama)

This is a great energizer breath. Beginners should practice Bellows Breath sitting down, but those who are more experienced in breathing practices could do it standing up. This practice is not recommended during pregnancy or for those with hypertension or panic disorder. Substitute with *Ujjayi* Breath (see page 41) for 1–3 minutes.

- To begin, take a few breaths in and out through your nose, noticing your belly expand on the inhale and contract on the exhale.

- Inhale a natural half-breath, then begin Bellows Breath by exhaling forcefully through your nose and inhaling at the same rate, which is quick—about one cycle per second. The inhale and exhale are even in tempo and intensity. Your body is still and straight except for the pumping action in your diaphragm.

- Begin with 10 rounds and rest for 3–5 natural breaths in between. Then work up to 20 rounds and then 30 rounds with the resting breaths in between. If you feel lightheaded or dizzy, relax and breathe naturally and stay with 10 pumps at a time for 3 rounds.

skull shining breath

(kapalabhati kriya)

This technique is a *kriya*, which is a breath practice that is used for clearing, cleansing and purifying, and revitalizing. It is most commonly done seated although can also be done standing up. This practice is not recommended during pregnancy or for those with hypertension or panic disorder. Substitute with *Ujjayi* Breath (see page 41) for 1–3 minutes.

- Place your hands on your belly or rest them on your legs. Inhale fully through your nose and exhale through your mouth.

- On your next inhale, stop short of a full breath and exhale through your nose with a forceful blow as your abdomen engages toward your navel.

- Let your inhale follow naturally. Focus on the exhale, which comes from the action of the belly pulling in. The inhale is a slower, natural reaction to the force of the exhale. Both breaths are done through the nose. It sounds a bit like a train chugging along or the piston of an engine.

- To start with, practice 3 rounds of 11 breaths with 2 or 3 natural breaths in between. You may eventually increase to 3 rounds of 27 breaths.

cooling breath
(sitali pranayama)

Cooling Breath is a natural air conditioner that is perfect for cooling a temper or mitigating a hot flash.

- Take a few deep breaths into your belly then form an "O" with your lips and slip your tongue through the opening, folding it to resemble a straw or tiny taquito.

- Wait until some saliva has formed and then breathe in through the "straw" (or bird's beak as the yogis saw it) drinking in the cool moisture.

- When you finish inhaling, close your lips and exhale completely through your nose.

- Continue with the breath for 3–5 minutes if possible.

ALTERNATIVE BREATH PRACTICE:
hissing breath (sitkari pranayama)

If you are not genetically predisposed to form a straw with your tongue, you can practice Hissing Breath, which is exactly the same practice but with a variation on the tongue position.

Gently press your teeth together and open your lips so your teeth are exposed. Your tongue is folded back so the underside presses the roof of your mouth, resembling a quesadilla.

Draw the moistened air in through the sides of your mouth and exhale through the nose.

bee breath
(bhramari pranayama)

This is wonderful for relieving stress and sends a healing vibration through the vocal chords and chest. It can be practiced seated, on a chair or the floor, or lying down.

- Place one hand on your heart and one hand on your belly.

- Inhale and as you exhale make a deep humming sound like a bee. Hum from the chest and belly more than from the lips. Let the "breath buzz" fade out naturally.

- Do not strain for the sound to last, rather let it softly and naturally fade in the way a buzz from a bee fades as it flies farther away from you.

lion's breath
(simhasana)

You may feel silly and awkward as you get used to roaring like a lion, but a little silly can go a long way to soothe an angry beast. Also, this breath tones the throat and neck (even lions appreciate a youthful appearance), strengthens the platysma muscle at the front of the throat, releases jaw tension, and activates the bandhas (energetic locks or binds).

- Choose your position: sit with big toes together and knees open, sit on your heels, or even lunge forward like a pouncing lion.

- Take a big inhale, and as you forcefully exhale spread your hands like giant paws with claws, press them down into your legs or the floor, and simultaneously stick your tongue out and roll your wide-open eyes toward your third eye (see page 142).

- Freeze for 20 seconds in the pose. Then relax and breathe normally. Repeat twice.

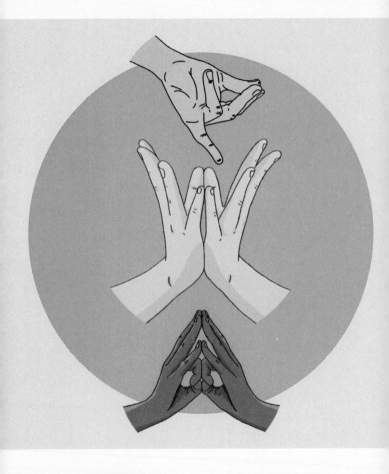

∞·∞·∞·∞·∞·∞·∞·∞·∞·∞·∞·∞·∞·∞

chapter three

mudras and meditations

Mudras are mainly positions that we take with
our hands in the same way we use the body to
take positions in yoga. They can be used on
their own, as part of a yoga or breath practice,
or to aid meditation.

∞·∞·∞·∞·∞·∞·∞·∞·∞·∞·∞·∞·∞·∞

how to mudra

I love thinking of mudra as a verb. To mudra or not to mudra? Well, since it literally breaks down to "bring forth delight," I say you'll never go wrong with a mudra! So let's go over a few helpful hints to get the most from your mudras. We will refer to the mudras by their Sanskrit name as is the more common practice.

MUDRA PREP 101

Like any other part of the body, the hands will enjoy a little TLC before launching into a position, so ideally, and if possible, spend a few moments rubbing the hands together vigorously, wiggle the fingers or flick them, and circle your wrists a few times in each direction. This can loosen the joints, increase the circulation, and stimulate the nadis (energy channels) for an increased effect.

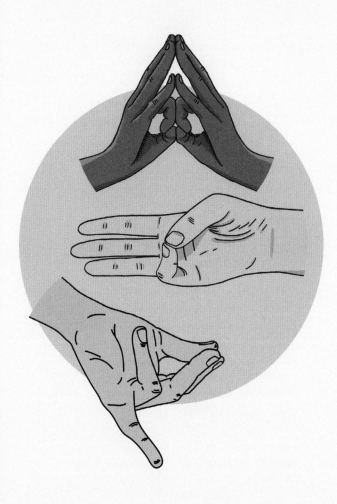

daily mudras

I always suggest a morning and/or night practice for all aspects of yoga, especially for breath practices, mudras, and meditation.

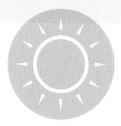

MORNING MUDRA

In the morning, we have cleared our emotional palette, released mental momentum, rested the body, and have a sense of rebirth. It's the perfect time to create a positive vibration by holding your attention on an intention that aligns your body, mind, and spirit to energetically design your day. A 10–20-minute breath and mudra practice in the morning will have a powerful and lasting effect throughout the day.

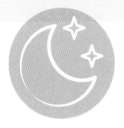

NIGHTTIME MUDRA

A few serene and reflective moments at the end of the day can cleanse and cure a million small ills. I highly recommend a 10–20-minute practice of chosen breath and mudra that appeals to you, offering up your day and letting go. The sweet moments will linger, the challenges be muted or handed over to the higher power for the night, and some grateful reflection can bring order to chaos. This ritual can make the difference between a deep peaceful sleep or a restless night still wrestling the demons of the day.

when to mudra

EMERGENCY MUDRAS

This is the prescription for on-the-spot mood adjustments. You may find yourself holding a mudra at your desk, in the doctor's or dentist's office, or on public transportation. You can carry this book with you for just such moments, or you may wish to familiarize yourself with a few "go-to" mudras.

With this style of mudra practice we are simply employing an excellent tool as a reminder that while we may not have control of the events outside of ourselves, we do have choices about how we react. If possible, hold the mudra for a minimum of 3 minutes with your attention in the present.

INTUITIVE MUDRAS

With these mudras, you are focusing on tuning in and centering yourself. Set aside time to practice. You can scroll through the book and choose what appeals to you in relation to this intention, or you can tune in and do an internal check, kindly asking your higher self,

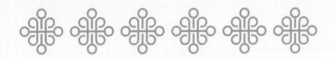

"What do I need today?"

For these mudras, I suggest holding for a minimum of 3 minutes up to 30 minutes once or twice a day, or following the instructions that correspond with the breaths.

THERAPEUTIC MUDRAS

For chronic or severe conditions, you will reap greater benefits if you approach the mudras with a healthy dose of discipline and think of them as natural medicine. Begin by holding the mudras for 3 minutes minimum, several times a day. Then, as your hands adjust and grow stronger and more flexible, you may find you can move to 3 times per day for 15 minutes.

If it's possible for you, you can even work your way up to holding the mudras for 45 minutes at a stretch. This may seem like a lot (and it is!) so don't fret if that's not possible—it's more important to practice frequently and consistently, especially with more challenging conditions.

mudras and meditation

Mudras are extremely helpful in beginning or maintaining a meditation practice as they act as an anchor for the restless mind, tethering it to the moment. It is not necessary to meditate formally while practicing mudras but you may find that you drop into a state of mindfulness with less mental effort when including the mudras.

JEWEL THOUGHTS

In Hindu and Buddhist texts, as well as various spiritual literature sources, the lotus flower is seen as representing human divinity (the jewel in the center) within the cosmos (the lotus flower). Although the practice of yoga itself requires no religious or spiritual affiliation and can be practiced by anyone of any background, it is by nature spiritual in that it serves as a path to enlightenment—the state of consciousness, or "beingness," in which we are aware and sensitive to the suffering, pain, and hardships of being human but live in a state of inner peace and bliss.

Like the jewel at the center of the lotus flower, jewel thoughts are the affirmative gems that nestle at the heart of each practice. They are the consolidated essence of each condition in its simplest, pure, positive form. You may discover that you resonate with them or you don't. You may find that they stimulate the desire to hatch your own jewel thought!

I have included jewel thoughts with the following mudras. If you choose to use them, you can place the book in front of you and refer to the jewel thought as offered while practicing your choice of mudra, or you can take a more concentrated approach by repeating the jewel thought silently or out loud until you have it firmly in your mind, before adopting the mudra position. The most essential component is that you allow yourself to truly feel the thought and embrace its meaning.

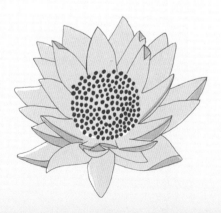

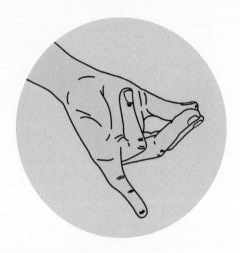

mahasirs mudra
(large head mudra)

This mudra helps you to enter a state of relaxation in which pressure and tension build-up may retreat and allow the healing life force called prana flow. It works wonders for headaches, and when combined with either the Alternate Nostril Breath (see page 48) or *Ujjayi* Breath (see page 41) for 10–30 rounds, you might make this your new over-the-counter headache cure!

- Touch your thumb, index, and middle fingers together.

- Fold your ring finger into your palm.

- Extend your pinky finger.

- Either do this with your free hand or both hands and rest the hands, palms up, on your thighs or knees.

JEWEL THOUGHT

I release all tension in body and mind. My mind is open and free. I am free.

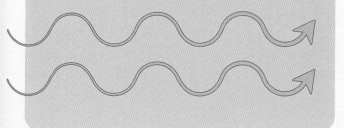

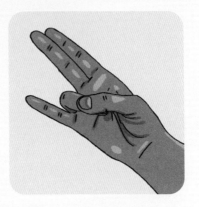

prithvi mudra
(earth mudra)

This mudra works by decreasing the element of fire energy (agni) and increasing the earth (kapha) element, which helps restore, rebuild, and prevent burnout—it's a replenishing mudra. It is also said to help with digestion and metabolism, and control hunger. It has a few variations and is sometimes called the Sun Mudra since it invokes fire energy. You can combine it with Skull Shining Breath (see page 51) or *Ujjayi* Breath (see page 41).

JEWEL THOUGHT

I am whole and complete.
I am filled with light and love.

- Place your hands, palms up, on your thighs, or hold up your hands with bent elbows at shoulder height.

- Bend your ring fingers on each hand into your palm.

- Press the thumbs into the ring fingers, holding them down.

- The index and middle fingers extend, touching each other.

- The pinky fingers extend.

pran mudra
(life-force mudra)

This "powerhouse mudra" has many applications. It stimulates the even flow of blood and prana in the body, which increases vitality when circulating freely through the whole system. That vitality is more than just physical energy; it's access to the vastness of cosmic consciousness and source energy that ignites the life force or prana. You can combine this mudra with Skull Shining Breath (see page 51) or Sun Breath (see page 44).

JEWEL THOUGHT

I am lit up with the creative life force of the universe.

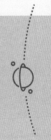

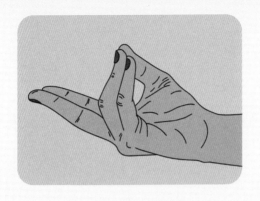

- Bring your thumbs, ring and pinky fingers together on each hand.

- Index and middle fingers are together and extended.

- Place your hands, palms up, on your thighs.

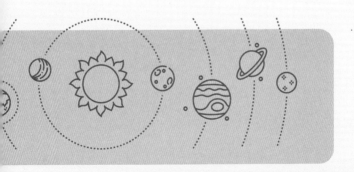

hansi mudra
(swan mudra)

This mudra moves the energy upward toward the heart and face to uplift the spirit. It also promotes feelings of courage and fearlessness, which are wonderful for anxious minds and battling feelings of loneliness or isolation. Pair it with Hissing Breath (see page 53) or Three-Part Breath (see page 42).

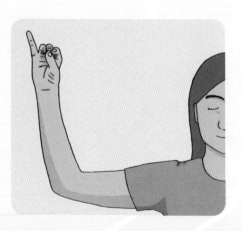

- Bring your thumbs, index, middle, and ring fingers together on each hand, pinky fingers extended.

- Either set the back of your hands on your thighs or hold both arms to the side at shoulder height, elbows bent, hands pointing upward.

JEWEL THOUGHT

I am uplifted,
happiness flows
to me and through me
as I glide through my life.

padmasana mudra
(lotus mudra)

This mudra is a symbol of purity and is connected to the heart chakra (see page 142). The lotus symbolizes our journey from dark to light as it travels from the murky river bed to the light of day, remaining clean, pure, and unsoiled despite the journey as it floats on the surface of the water. You can pair it with *Ujjayi* Breath (see page 41).

JEWEL THOUGHT

I am open, pure,
and filled with love.

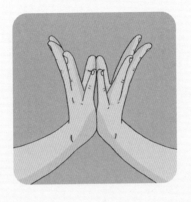

- Place the hands in front of the heart center with the heels of the hands touching.

- Bring the tips of the pinky fingers and thumbs to touch.

- Fan the other fingers open like a fully bloomed lotus flower.

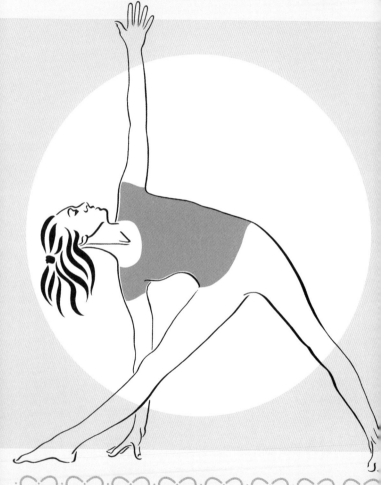

chapter four

for the body:
top to bottom

In this section, we will use asanas (poses) along with
mudras (hand gestures) and pranayama
(breathing techniques) to relieve many common
physical concerns. Come to your practice from a
place of acceptance and curiosity whenever
possible. Yoga is goal-oriented, but no goal is as
accentuated as that of staying present with "what
is." Whatever your hopes may be for alleviating the
condition you find yourself in, remain open to the
bounty of possibilities that may await you.

headache

Headaches may ambush us for a variety of reasons, but according to the Mayo Clinic, the biggest contributor is stress! When we calm the body and mind, we soothe the highly charged nervous system, helping to restore harmony and peace of mind, which may decrease tension and pain. The best way to treat a headache is with *Ujjayi* Breath (see page 41) combined with *Mahasirs Mudra* (see page 66), Downward Dog (see page 22), or Legs up the Wall.

LEGS UP THE WALL (OR INVERTED ACTION)
(VIPARITA KARANI)

- Try visualizing a beautiful, serene lake and imagine your breath as a gentle breeze that does not disturb the surface of the water.

- Sit with your left hip against the wall. You can be on the floor or on a firm blanket or bolster. Put your weight onto your hands and arms as you swing your legs up the wall until you can lie back on the floor.

- Your lower back should be on the bolster or floor. If your hamstrings or back feel strained or you are having to make an effort to hold the pose, move yourself a few inches away from the wall and let your legs rest on an incline. You may also find it more comfortable to open the legs into a slight V shape.

- Hold for 5–10 minutes with your focus on the gentle rise and fall of your breath.

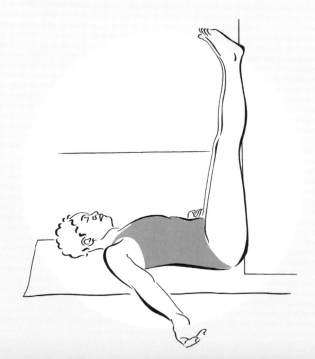

pain in the neck

When you are suffering from a sore or stiff neck, it can be hard to ignore it. After all, your neck supports your head and the ability to turn your head is pretty crucial. Whether you've slept yourself into a predicament, are suffering from a sudden spasm, or have chronic neck pain, try easing it with gentle neck stretches and rolls while in *Sukhasana* (see page 16). You could also try Child's Pose (see page 24), elevating your head using a block or stack of books until it feels comfortable, or a variation on Bridge Pose.

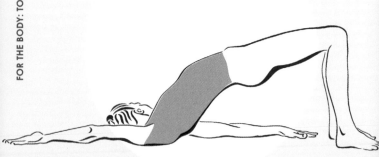

BRIDGE POSE VARIATION
(SETU BANDHASANA)

- Come into Bridge Pose (see page 136) by lying on your back and bending your knees so that your feet are directly under your knees and parallel to each other. Rest your arms by your sides and position your face toward the ceiling with the back of your neck long. Do not jut your chin upward.

- On an inhale, lift up your hips and take your right arm all the way back behind you so that the back of your hand touches the floor. At the same time, slowly roll your head to the left, away from your arm.

- On your exhale, bring your hips down and your arm back by your side as your head returns to center.

- Repeat on the other side to complete one cycle. Do 4–6 cycles.

- Move slowly and synchronize your movements to your breath. Think of this as a dry-land backstroke and get into a rhythm as you would while swimming.

tight throat

The fifth chakra, called *Vishuddha* (see page 142), is located in the throat and is our link to expressing ourselves. When the voice feels constricted or compromised, or we lose it, feelings of frustration, isolation, and even depression may soon follow. However, as we know, yoga lowers stress levels and promotes relaxation, and these beneficial effects may be felt in the throat just like anywhere else. Try Bee Breath (see page 54) or Supported Fish.

SUPPORTED FISH
(SALAMBA MATSYASANA)

- Position a bolster, rolled-up blanket, or block where your shoulder blades will be when you lie on the floor.

- From *Dandasana* (see page 12), lower yourself onto your set-up, and use your hands to press your thighs down and toward your feet. If you find your neck needs more support or your head needs some height, place another rolled-up blanket or towel behind your neck or under your head. Your arms may be out to the side, bent at the elbows, palms up.

- Once you are in the pose, close your eyes and take your attention to your throat chakra. If you are able and so inclined, try to visualize your favorite version of turquoise at your throat center—it could be a body of water or a gemstone, or just a free-floating color—and take a few breaths. If this is difficult for you, don't fret, just focus on the physical center of your throat.

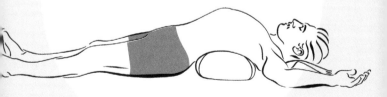

shoulder tension

Ever feel like you have too much on your shoulders? Or find yourself flinching in traffic? Responsibility has a way of settling into and onto the shoulders. Whatever the reason may be, the chronic shrug position can be painful and disrupt your happy flow. Lighten your load with Standing Forward Fold (see page 20) with your hands clasped behind your back or Eagle Arms.

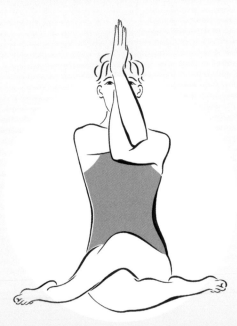

EAGLE ARMS

(GARUDASANA ARMS)

- Come to hands and knees and place your left knee behind your right, sitting back between your feet with the right knee stacked on top of the left. Place your feet in line with each other on either side of your hips.

- As you inhale, stretch your arms wide at shoulder height with your palms facing up. Hold there with the arms outstretched for 3 breaths. Concentrate on rotating the inner arms up toward the sky and keeping the palms wide and facing directly up.

- On an exhale, wrap your arms with the left arm over the right, bend your elbows, and face the back of the hands toward each other. Your elbows should be parallel to the floor and chest high.

- Move your left hand to the left and your right hand to the right until your right pinky passes your left thumb, and place the fingers of your right hand into the palm of your left as much as is possible for you.

- Take 5 deep breaths here, gazing directly in front of you, and then slowly release the pose. Let your arms hang by your sides and relax for a few moments before repeating on the other side.

upper back

The upper back (thoracic spine) can morph into a block of ice seemingly overnight. It protects the vital organs in the chest by being a stable and less flexible point in the spine, but when our modern lives lead us to spend hours hunched over a desk or table, it's time to sit up (literally) and take notice. You can find relief with the Cat Cow.

CAT COW (OR CROOKED OR CHURNING WHEEL)
(CHAKRAVAKASANA)

- Begin on all fours in the Tabletop Pose (see page 18) with hands under shoulders and knees under hips.

- Relax your belly and soften the upper back while opening the chest and inhaling. Keep your shoulders back from your ears and tilt your head up slightly but not so much that you are crunching your cervical spine by collapsing your head onto your neck. Take care not to overarch your lower back, but rather concentrate on opening the chest and relaxing the abdomen. This is Cow Pose (A).

- As you begin to exhale, move into Cat Pose (think scary Halloween cat) by tightening your abdominals and rounding your spine up toward the ceiling. Push into the earth with your hands, shins, and knees and let your head hang down (B).

- In both positions your arms stay straight. Practice 5–10 rounds, then rest in Child's Pose (see page 24).

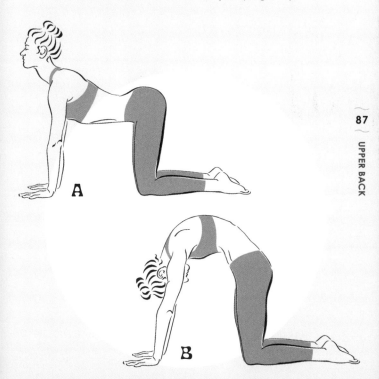

tight chest

When we collapse the chest from chronic slouching, the muscles in the chest wall get tight and this restricts the flow of blood and oxygen, leaving us a little deflated in body and spirit. A wonderful way to expand your physical heart center and boost your mood is to practice Supported Fish (see page 82) or Cobra Pose.

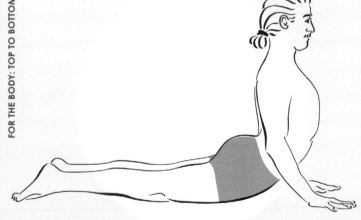

COBRA POSE
(BHUJANGASANA)

- Lie flat on the floor with your forehead on the ground and your hands, pointing forward, right beneath your shoulders, elbows bent backward.

- Lengthen your legs behind you, extending directly out from your hips, and place all ten toenails on the floor.

- Rooting into your hips and pelvis, inhale as you rise up like a cobra slowly emerging to fan its chest. Keep firm pressure into the floor from your pelvis to your feet, because this is the foundation from which you can open your chest.

- It is not necessary to straighten your arms, and for some people not desirable because it can compromise the lower back. So your arms may be bent or straight, depending on how comfortable your low back feels.

- Seek to open your chest and strengthen your upper back muscles by focusing on the breath and staying tuned in to your sensations. Hold for 3–5 breaths, exhaling as you come down. Repeat 3 times.

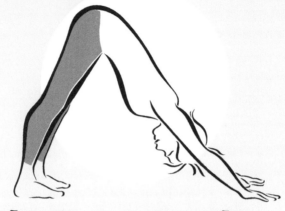

middle back pain

Middle back pain tends to get lost until it has reached fever pitch and demands to be noticed! It may flare up because of strain or injury, prolonged hours of sitting, or what I like to call "losing the jelly in your doughnut." The pain may be localized or spread into buttocks and legs. Fortunately, my personal and professional experience has shown that tremendous improvement can be achieved through yoga! The dynamic duo of strengthening and fostering flexibility comes into play again here. You can find relief with the Downward Dog Pose (see page 22) or Child's Pose (see page 24).

lower back pain

Every part of the world shares the affliction of back pain by the millions. Of those millions many are suffering chronically, which is widely considered to be three months or longer. The much better news is that yoga really helps and in many cases heals. We know that injury and long hours at a desk or behind the wheel take their toll on the body and in particular the lower back. Back pain also tends to flare up when stress levels are at their peak. So the yoga way would be to kill it (or let's say love it) with kindness. That means strengthen, stretch with the Supine Twist (see page 27), and relax. Remember, consistency is key for something chronic, but every little bit does count, so do what you can, when you can, and appreciate yourself for your effort!

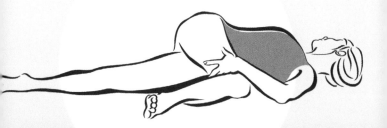

lady trouble

If irritability, mood swings, bloating, muscle pain, and exhaustion are part of your monthly excursion into all things female, and you are hungry for an exit, a yoga practice may be your golden key to freedom. While it is best (always) to make space for a regular yoga practice to achieve maximum benefits, taking 15 minutes out of your day can work wonders. Turn the lights down, turn the phone off, light a candle if you have one near, and reclaim the beauty of your femininity with Legs up the Wall (see page 78).

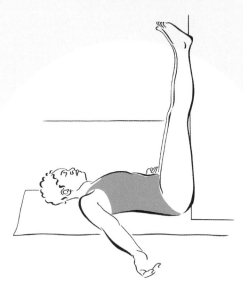

menopause

Ah, the price we may pay to enter the golden gates of wisdom. If you have ever felt as though you have been catapulted into a furnace or that your fuse is not only too short but barely even there, you know the prickly edge of menopause. Disrupted sleep, mental fog, sadness, and despair are just a few more symptoms. However, there are many beautiful aspects of the aging process, and when we allow ourselves to be present through the changing terrain, we notice the subtle, and often not so subtle, treasures that are revealed.

While a consistent yoga practice can certainly keep our bones dense, muscles strong, and lungs healthy, it may be the sweetness of a deepening compassion for ourselves and all things, which arises from your practice, that becomes the most healing element of all.

To help relieve symptoms of menopause, try the Bridge Pose (see page 136), which is a restorative heart opener, or Cooling Breath (see page 52), perfect for those hot flashes.

bloating

Bloating can occur from what we eat, the way we eat (too much and too fast), and even stress and anxiety, which inhibit digestion. A yoga practice can improve digestion by the way the organs are manipulated in the poses as well as by reducing overall anxiety. Try the Hugging Knees to Chest pose (see page 19), Supine Twist (see page 27), or Half Lord of the Fishes.

HALF LORD OF THE FISHES
(ARDHA MATSYENDRASANA)

- Sit on the floor with your legs out in front of you. If this already feels like trouble, sit up on a folded blanket to support your lower back.

- Bend your knees so that your feet are on the floor, and slide your right leg under your left. Your right thigh will be on the floor and your left foot will be squarely on the ground.

- Hug your left knee to help elongate your spine. Take your right arm up in the air, as if you were picking the best piece of fruit from the top of the tree, then bend your elbow and bring it down outside of your left knee, as if you were going to take a bite. Keep the hand active.

- Meanwhile, take your left arm back behind you and press on the floor with your fingertips or palm. If you find it difficult to reach the floor, place a block or books underneath your palm until you can sit comfortably straight.

- When you inhale, let your abdomen expand as much as it can, and when you exhale, squeeze your navel in toward your spine. Don't force the breath; stay relaxed and alert, concentrating on a full, even breath.

- Hold for 4–7 breaths, then repeat on the other side.

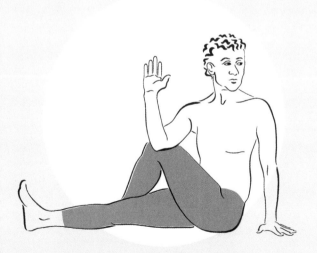

tight hips

In my experience, the most frequently requested of all yoga positions are those that open the hips. It is the physical location of the the second chakra, *Svadhisthana* (see page 142), the energy center for emotions, and the pelvis is the perfect bowl-like shape to hold them. Ease the tension with Butterfly Pose (also known as Cobbler's Pose) or One-legged King Pigeon (see page 112).

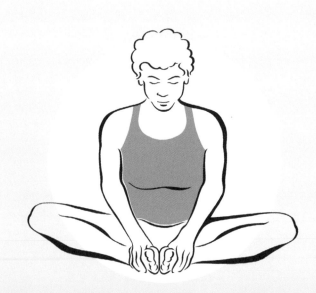

BUTTERFLY POSE (OR COBBLER'S POSE)
(BADDHA KONASANA)

- In a seated position, bring the soles of your feet together with your knees out to the sides. Wrap your index and middle fingers around your two big toes in yogi toelock and lengthen up through your spine.

- Press your feet firmly together with your toes spread apart so you feel your inner thighs wake up, and on an exhale extend forward as far as you can without rounding your back too dramatically.

- From here you may wish to take your hands out in front of you or onto some blocks or books. Placing the hands in front of you can add a stretch for the shoulders and brings a restorative flavor to the pose. If you stay holding your toes, be sure to curl your big toes slightly in so they don't feel overstretched.

- Stay for 1–5 minutes enjoying the sensation of your breath slowly opening and closing the imaginary wings on your back like a butterfly.

thighs and knees

Knees are the precious shock absorbers that bear the brunt of much of our life experience. If through injury, arthritis, or developmental issues your knees are not pleased, take heart—there is hope. In the case of the knees, what strengthens often heals, but a fair dose of stretch for the quadriceps is a main ingredient. Strengthen and stretch with Chair Pose or Triangle Pose (see page 100).

CHAIR POSE
(UTKATASANA)

- Start in *Tadasana* (see page 14) with the feet together and parallel to each other, spine straight, and kneecaps lifted. You may be more comfortable with your heels slightly apart and toes touching. Try both ways and see which fits.

- Bend the knees and sweep the arms straight up in front of you until your biceps are by your ears.

- Rock into your heels a bit. Spread your toes and place them down on the mat with space between each toe. Keep the weight in the heels while still pressing into the balls of the feet. Let your shoulders drop away from your ears (avoid the shrug position) and keep the arms vibrantly straight.

- Contract your navel toward your spine to protect the back. You should have a natural and comfortable curve in your lumbar spine, but not an exaggerated arch.

- Hold for 5 breaths, then push into the earth with strong legs and stand up in *Tadasana*. Repeat 3–5 times.

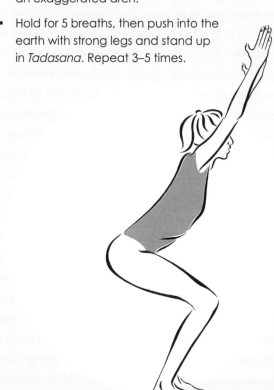

TRIANGLE POSE
(TRIKONASANA)

- Start in *Tadasana* (see page 14), place your hands on your hips, and step your feet wide apart (approximately 4 feet/1.25 meters).

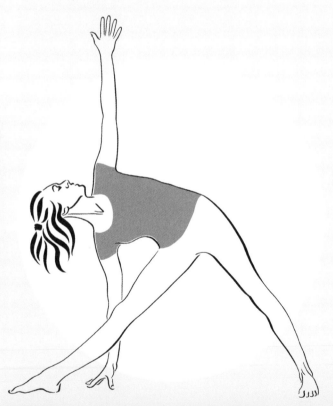

- Turn your left heel to the left slightly and your right foot 90 degrees to the right. Stretch your arms out to the sides at shoulder height with the palms facing down.

- As you inhale, reach out over your right toe tips with your right hand and extend your torso out over the right leg. Exhale and place your right hand on your leg, a block, or the floor. You can have the hand inside or outside of the right foot, as long as you are able to keep your right hand under your right shoulder and extend both sides of your waist toward the right.

- Engage your thighs and track your right knee over your shin bone and down to your second right toe. Your left arm is directly over your left shoulder and your focus point (see page 14) is your left thumb. If possible, don't bend the neck to the side, but keep it extending directly out from your spine.

- Hold for 2–5 breaths, come up with a strong core and legs, and repeat on the other side.

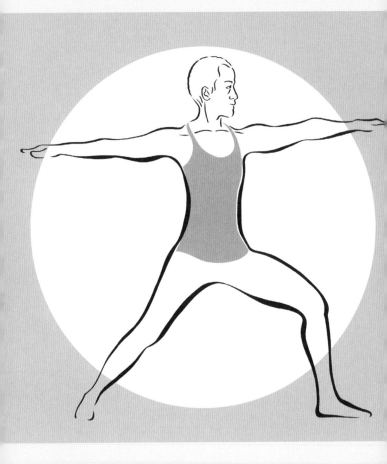

chapter 5

for the mind: who is running this show?

The mind can be viewed as a wild and majestic horse that simply needs to be loved (not broken) into calmness so that its own reckless energy doesn't consume it. This section encourages the use of asanas, breath, and meditation to relax the mind into the eternally present moment from which all is possible, and where all exists.

anxiety

Situational anxiety is a normal part of life, but it can become a tidal wave with an extreme undertow, leaving you with inner turmoil, muscular tension, mental exhaustion, and general nervousness. Yoga works beautifully for assuaging anxious moments in life. Find relief with *Hansi Mudra* (see page 72), Three Part Breath (see page 42), or balancing poses like Tree Pose.

TREE POSE
(VRKSASANA)

- Stand in *Tadasana* (see page 14) and choose a focus point (see page 14). Feel all four corners of each foot placed evenly and firmly upon the earth.

- Bring your hands to your hips and shift your weight to the right foot. Lift your left leg, bending the knee until you can reach down for your ankle without bending over too significantly.

- Once you have grasped your ankle, place it on the upper inner right thigh with your toes pointing toward the floor. Keep pressing your inner right foot down to stay rooted. Rotate your inner left thigh out as much as you can to open that left hip.

- Make the *Atmanjali Mudra* (pictured, see page 128) or *Hakini Mudra* (see page 108) and hold directly in front of your heart. The *Atmanjali Mudra* directs the breath or energy into the heart space and allows the union of the body with the cosmic energy, helping to bring stability to the mind, while the *Hakini Mudra* helps us connect to the third eye (see page 142), developing our intuition, clarity, and calm.

- Stay for 5–10 breaths or until you feel the urge to move, and release into *Tadasana* before you switch sides.

fear

In those moments when we are unable to embrace the unpredictable nature of life, fear can set in. There are many things to fear, but if we can master a few techniques, we have a better chance of feeling empowered to choose in which direction to go and where to put our focus. Warm up with 5 rounds of Sun Salutations (see page 30) before practicing your Bellows Breath (see page 50) or Warrior II.

WARRIOR II
(VIRABHADRASANA II)

- From *Tadasana* (see page 14), step your feet wide apart and extend your arms at shoulder height. Your ankles should line up under your wrists.

- Turn your left foot in on a 30-degree angle with your toes facing right. Turn your right foot out to face directly away from your body and pointing forward. Keep your spine upright, with your chest directly over your belly button and your hips square.

- On an exhale, bend the right knee slowly while maintaining contact with the floor through the left heel. Make sure your right knee tracks over the second toe of your foot.

- Set your focus point (see page 14) over the middle finger of your right hand. Relax your shoulders but keep the arms extended. Engage your abdominals and hold for 3–5 breaths.

- On an inhale, lift out of the pose and rest your hands on your hips. Turn your feet to the other side and repeat.

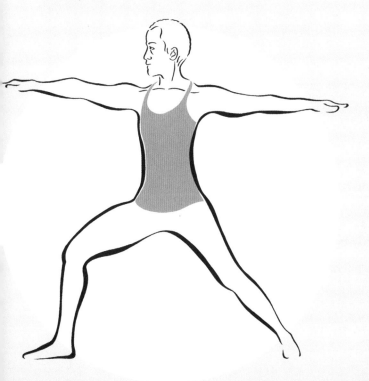

lack of focus

It can happen anytime, anywhere, and often at the worst possible moment. Your mind wanders in every direction but where you need it to stay right now. As stated by the yogic sage Patanjali in the Yoga Sutras, "Yoga chitta vritti nirodha," which translates as, "Yoga is the reduction of fluctuations of the mind." Wrangle that magnificent mind of yours with Warrior II (see page 106). Alternate Nostril Breath (see page 48) is also great for this, or try simple Breath Awareness (see page 39) while adopting *Hakini Mudra*, which generates power to rule over a restless mind. Before you begin, bring to mind the jewel thought below as an intention for your practice.

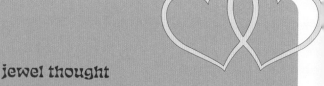

jewel thought
I am steady and awake.
My mind is strong and clear.

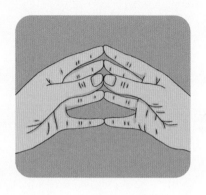

HAKINI MUDRA
(POWER OR RULE MUDRA)

- Bring the fingertips of the right hand to touch the fingertips of the left hand.

- Your elbows are bent and your hands are in front of your ribcage or where it feels natural.

- Use a slight pressure coming from your arms to press the fingertips together.

- Use a sand timer, clock, or inner clock to hold the mudra while focusing on the breath for 3 minutes minimum.

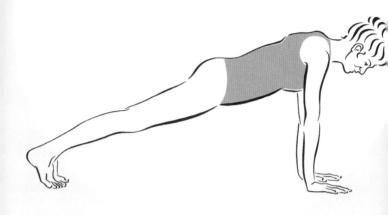

procrastination

Even for those who are gifted at pulling through at the eleventh hour, procrastination has heavy repercussions on the body, mind, and spirit. Poses that activate the solar plexus, our core chakra (see page 142), help to empower and revitalize us to get over mental barriers. Try Downward Dog (see page 22) or Plank Pose.

PLANK POSE
(UTTHITA CHATURANGA DANDASANA)

- You can come into Plank from Downward Dog or from the floor. To come into the pose from the floor, start in Tabletop Pose (see page 18) with your hands under your shoulders and step one leg back at a time.

- If starting from Downward Dog, simply lift up onto the balls of your feet and roll your torso forward, like a wave, while pulling your belly button in toward your spine. Your hands may not line up under your wrists (where we want them), in which case you will need to shift a little to place them properly. The balls of your feet should be under your heels and hip-width apart.

- Soften your upper back so that it "melts" between your shoulder blades. Engage your abdominals and hug your triceps toward each other, keeping the shoulders moving away from your ears. The back of your head remains in line with your spine. Your body should slope gently from your shoulders to your hips to your heels, resembling a piece of wood that is on a slight incline.

- Hold Plank for 3–5 breaths for 3 rounds. Rest either in Downward Dog or Child's Pose (see page 24) in between each round.

apathy

Apathy can be the result of a creative or romantic dry spell, or erupt in the wake of overwhelming news or a series of challenging events. Yoga encourages the movement of prana (life force) and functions as an antidote to apathy. Get your blood flowing with Sun Salutations (see page 30), then practice your Sun Breath (see page 44), *Pran Mudra* (see page 70), or One-legged King Pigeon Pose.

ONE-LEGGED KING PIGEON
(EKA PADA RAJAKAPOTASANA)

- From Butterfly Pose (see page 96), swing your right leg behind you and square your hips.

- Try to move your left leg into a position that is parallel to the front edge of your yoga mat if you are using one. It should resemble a straight horizontal line with your foot flexed.

- If this puts a strain on your knee, draw the foot nearer to your pelvis and release the flex. You may want to put a blanket under your left hip if you are sinking to that side and losing the square of your hips.

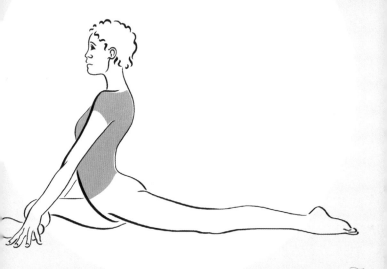

- Extend your back leg straight out from the hip and press your toenails into the floor. Your foot should be centered, not sickled.

- You can stay here propped up on your hands, or you can walk your hands forward into a comfortable "pigeon nap" as long as you maintain the alignment of your hips and legs.

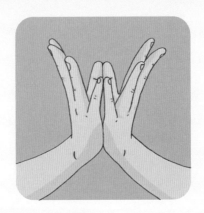

the blues

Falling somewhere between sorrow and apathy and shuffling on the edge of depression, the blues may be excellent fodder for some of our favorite pieces of music and art, but the reality of being in a blue rut is nowhere near as romantic as it may sound.

Balancing poses are effective for pulling us out of the past and into the now—try it yourself with the Tree Pose (see page 104). You can then add *Padmasana Mudra* (Lotus Mudra, see page 74) to your Tree Pose. The lotus flower symbolizes delight: it grows in the murky, dense goo at the bottom of the lake or river and moves unerringly toward the light for a year before bursting to the surface in all its

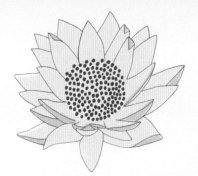

resonance and glory, unstained by its grimy beginnings. If you wish, adopt the jewel thought below while in this pose.

Alternatively, try Downward Dog (see page 22)—getting your feet over your head will shake things up in all the right ways! Similarly, Skull Shining Breath (see page 51) is an excellent breath practice for the blues because it is revitalizing.

jewel thought
I am open, pure, and filled with love.

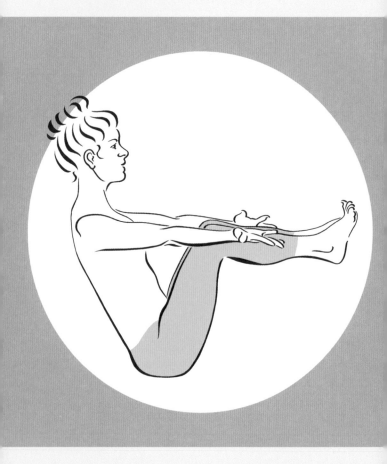

chapter 6

for the spirit: bring your heartsong to life

It is easy to believe in only what we can see or physically feel. The body is right there, made of blood, flesh, and bone. We know when we are hurt because there is visible evidence. The spirit speaks in a language no less dynamic, but one that requires a deft ear and willing mind to translate. We will use the practice of yoga to connect with, to listen to, and even to request a higher awareness of what it is that animates us and brings our heartsong to life.

love

When we turn our attention to love in any form, it shifts our immediate experience. Focusing on what and whom we love can color our perceptions of the day, or even our lives, almost instantaneously. The heart, which is the energetic center for the feeling of love, is remarkably resilient and tenacious both physically and emotionally. The desire to give and receive love is as mighty as this muscular organ's ability to continuously pump blood through the body. Let's get our love on with this guided meditation.

SUPPORTED FISH WITH GUIDED MEDITATION
(SALAMBA MATSYASANA)

- Come into Supported Fish (see page 82). If you can do so while pressing your feet against a wall, so much the better, but it's not essential. The aim is to have an earthy, grounded feeling so that you feel safe and supported to open through the heart center. Visualize the way a fish leaps out of the water and allow that freedom and lightness to come into your chest as you stay anchored through your legs.

- Once you are comfortably in the pose, close your eyes and turn your attention to your breath. Feel it coming into your heart center and visualize a flower bud there, perhaps a lotus flower or any that you love. With each gentle inhale, see the petals begin to open. With each exhale, relax into the slow unfolding of the flower.

- Continue with this visualization until the flower is fully bloomed in the center of your chest. Then inhale in three parts, or "sniffs," drawing in the sweetness of the moment, and exhale all tension from body and mind through an open mouth. Do this 3 times, then rest and breathe naturally.

- Leave the pose when you are ready, easing onto one side, bending your knees, and rolling up to a seated position or pushing down with your hands and sitting up with bent knees. Take a few moments to feel the effects of your renewed and open heart.

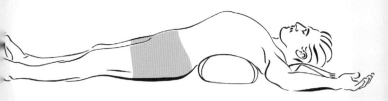

joy

The physical center for joy is the solar plexus (see page 142). Connecting to your core by strengthening and stretching can activate feelings of confidence and worthiness, and therefore nurture your capacity for joy. When you are centered from within and accepting of yourself, you can more easily access joy and have your "fun in the sun." Warm up with a few rounds of Sun Salutations (see page 30) before trying Boat Pose, perfect for evoking your sunny nature.

BOAT POSE
(NAVASANA)

- From a sitting position, bend your knees and place your feet on the floor.

- Rock back, supporting yourself with your hands, and point your feet so that just your toes touch the floor.

- Lift your feet off the floor, keeping your knees bent, then extend your feet so that they are at the same height as your knees. Point your toes, or flex the balls of your feet and fan your toes.

- Lift and extend your arms to either side of your legs, engaging your abdominal muscles. Keep your spine straight and your chest lifted. If you feel good here, continue to extend your legs to straight. If you have back pain, or it is too difficult for any reason, bend the knees again. You may also feel better clasping your hands behind your knees.

- Take 3–5 breaths, then come down, cross your legs, and, sitting tall, lift the arms to shoulder height and bend the elbows. With your hands, take the Mudra for Happiness by making peace-sign fingers, holding the ring and pinky fingers in with your thumb.

- Take 3–5 breaths and then return to the Boat one more time, finishing with the Mudra for Happiness, holding it for 1–3 minutes.

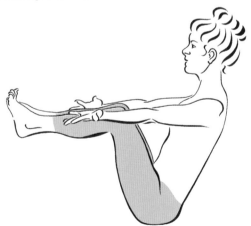

peace

To catch a ride on the peace train, we need to employ the understanding that it is not external events or situations that dictate our inner state of being— although life can throw us many a major doozy, for sure. Rather, our inner reality affects our perception of the outer reality. When we use the yogic tools of asana, pranayama, and meditation, we can mute knee-jerk reactions that often arise out of fear, stay in the moment, and actively practice peace.

Try it yourself with a variation of Butterfly Pose (see page 96), in which you rest your head on a block between your knees to de-stimulate the brain and activate the third eye (see page 142), or practice the Sphinx, a very calming and gently uplifting pose.

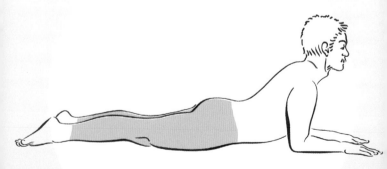

SPHINX POSE
(SALAMBA BHUJANGASANA)

- Lie on your belly and prop yourself up on your forearms.

- Place your elbows directly under your shoulders and spread your fingers wide, hands aligned with elbows and pressed into the floor. Your legs should extend straight back behind you with your toenails on the floor.

- Press the legs down as if imprinting them in sand, and slightly engage your lower belly.

- Pressing into the arms, slide your chest slightly forward and up. Your focus point (see page 14) is directly in front of you, with your chin level with the ground.

- Hold for 5–10 breaths, then rest by releasing down onto your belly, turning your toes out, and letting your heels fall in. If this feels very unnatural to you and uncomfortable, switch it around (toes in, heels out).

- Cross your arms so that your fingertips come near your elbows, and place your forehead on your forearms.

acceptance

Ironically, when we seek change, that's often the time when it may appear to be most elusive. This is where acceptance can be a deceptively active choice. If we can become more comfortable with the natural and dynamic law that life is always changing and so are we, we can lean into the flow of change and become inspired by possibility and the opportunity to grow—and to grow is our ultimate true nature. Practice your acceptance with the following challenge.

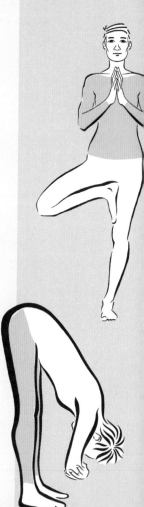

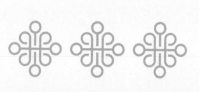

PICK YOUR POSE

Here you are going to choose a pose that is particularly challenging, whether that's because you're the type who "can't sit still", struggle with balance, or because of those pesky hips, crunchy shoulders, or stubborn hamstrings.

- Do a proper warm-up if necessary (see page 30).

- Get in your pose, hold it, breathe, and practice not resisting. That means physically not struggling or fidgeting and mentally not engaging in distracting commentary and opinions. Instead, focus on breathing and being present. If your mind is like a tiger in a cage, say to yourself, "This is what's happening," and then come back to the sound and feeling of your breath.

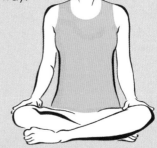

- Practice acceptance and observe if you feel your body and mind shift, release, transform. Even a little bit of acceptance can go a long way.

creativity

You don't need to be a professional, or even fledgling, artist to desire some spark in the arena of creativity. The sacral chakra (see page 142), located in the hips, is the energetic center for both creativity and pleasure, and it's no coincidence that these emanate from the same place. So let's loosen up the stuck energy in the hips with Swirling Butterfly and let that river of creativity flow! An alternative to this pose is Three-part Breath (see page 42), which is grounding, relaxing, and perfect for opening yourself to inspiration.

SWIRLING BUTTERFLY POSE
(BADDHA KONASANA)

- Sit on the floor in Butterfly Pose (see page 96), spine straight, knees out to the sides, and the soles of your feet together.

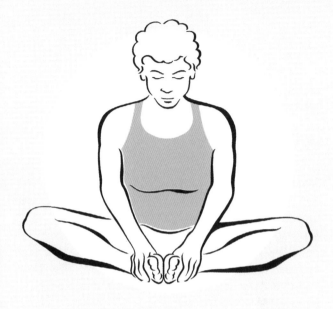

- Hold your ankles and move your body in circles, beginning clockwise. As you move toward your feet, inhale and let your belly expand. As you move your torso away from your feet, exhale and contract your belly.

- Swirl for 8 circles in each direction. When finished, hold Butterfly Pose for 5 more breaths, relaxing your belly.

appreciation and gratitude

Gratitude is taking the time to honor who and what we hold dear and to count our blessings. Appreciation has its own nuance. There is almost nothing as life-shifting as stopping in your tracks to appreciate. It can take a dark mood and bring in the light in a heartbeat. Sometimes the feelings of appreciation come effortlessly, but there are moments when we must remember and practice being receptive.

When we do endeavor consciously to live in a space of appreciation and gratitude, it can soften bad news, hard moments, and scary times and open our hearts and minds to the bounty of love and exquisiteness that surrounds us. Take a moment to appreciate your life with Thunderbolt Pose with *Atmanjali Mudra* or the Reverse Warrior (see page 130).

THUNDERBOLT POSE WITH ATMANJALI MUDRA
(VAJRASANA WITH REVERENCE TO THE HEART MUDRA)

- Sit on your shins with your sitting bones on the soles of your feet. This is Thunderbolt Pose.

- Bring your hands together in front of your heart center, but not touching the body. The fingers and base of the palms should touch each other but keep an open space in the center of the palms, enough to hold a small butterfly safely. This is *Atmanjali Mudra*.

- Lean a few inches forward with the head bowed. This position allows the heart energy to pour right into the hands, and softens the ego to submerge into a state of deep, peaceful gratitude. Stay as long as you like with easy breaths.

REVERSE WARRIOR
(VIPARITA VIRABHADRASANA)

- Before practicing the following sequence, I suggest that you do 5–10 rounds of Sun Salutations (see page 30) as a warm-up.

- From *Tadasana* (see page 14), come into Warrior II (see page 106), leading with your left leg. Hold for 3 breaths.

- Turn your palms up, and notice your heart lift and open. Inhale and lengthen upward through the crown of your head, making your spine long.

- Reach back with your right hand and place the palm on your right thigh. Stretch your left arm up to the sky and then arch back, with your left bicep a few inches from your left ear.

- You can stay facing to the side, or, if your back allows, you can twist your face and chest upward. Avoid putting pressure on the right leg, but rather keep a light touch with the palm and let the legs do the work. Like a tree, grow roots through your feet and let your heart open like a flower.

- Hold for 3–5 breaths and repeat on the other side.

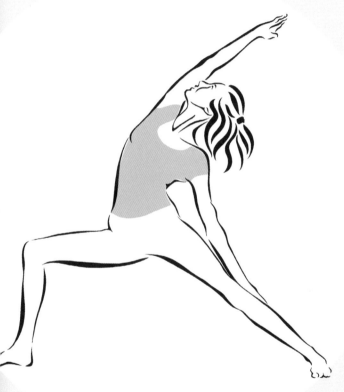

abundance

When we think of abundance in only practical, material terms, we tend to focus on the having rather than the being, which turns our attention to lack and fear of loss. When we touch upon the infinite nature of abundance, we unlock the potential to understand that there is never a scarcity of anything. Fear and clinging cut off our ability to flow, create, and receive. Let's tap into acknowledging all that is abundant here and now with Upward Plank Pose.

UPWARD PLANK POSE
(PURVOTTANASANA)

- Before beginning this sequence, I suggest that you do 5–10 rounds of Sun Salutations (see page 30) as a warm-up.

- To start, sit on the floor in *Dandasana* (see page 12).

- Place your hands 6–8 inches (15–20 centimeters) behind you, fingers still facing forward, and lean back.

- Point your toes, engage your legs, and push into the floor with your hands as you lift your hips and torso.

Squeeze the legs together and reach for the floor with your toes. Slowly, keeping your neck long, extend your head back.

- Breathe here, imagining all the bounty and abundance in your life sitting right on your abdomen like a table set for a feast. Keep your chest high, heart open, and breath steady for 3–5 breaths.

- Come down and rest in the Hugging Knees to Chest pose (see page 19).

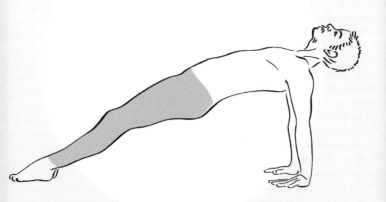

balance

Balance, like juggling, is a dynamic act. The urge is to over-organize our lives into a rigid idea of balance, but this can then overwhelm us. However, even with endless demands and responsibilities, we can artfully practice catching the balls with a smile. When we do fall, or drop the ball, we can display a sense of humor and move on.

Practice staying spontaneous, flexible, and connected to NOW with Alternate Nostril Breathing (see page 48), a technique that clears the two main energy channels of the body and results in greater energy and focus, or with the following variation on Tree Pose. If you wish, adopt the jewel thought below while in this pose.

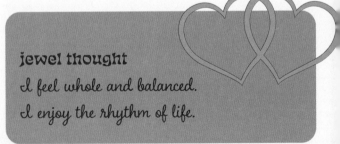

jewel thought
I feel whole and balanced.
I enjoy the rhythm of life.

TREE POSE VARIATION
(VRKSASANA)

- Get into Tree Pose (see page 104).

- When stable, position your hands in *Anjali Mudra* (palms and fingers pressed together like you're praying) at heart center.

- Close your eyes and move your gaze within. We tend to rely on our vision for much of our balance in the world, both physically and emotionally, by responding to external stimuli and reacting to what we see. When we let go of finding our footing based on what is surrounding us, we naturally drop into an inner center. While it may feel much less stable or sure-footed, the practice here is to relax into the wobble and sway, rather than to cling to the pose or rigid mindset. Finding balance can often come from being willing to let go and even fall.

- Find your edge in the pose, that turning point where holding on and letting go meet, like the sun passing the moon on its way to dawn.

energy

Energy—something we are born with in abundance and tend to appreciate and long for much more as we grow older. Fortunately, yoga can not only increase our energy but also balance it, so that we avoid those mysterious peaks and valleys and ease into a sustained groove of flowing life force.

Practice Skull Shining Breath (see page 51), which purifies the frontal brain, oxygenates the blood, and clears the mind, or Bridge Pose, a restorative heart opener that is wonderful for the mood, back, and lungs.

BRIDGE POSE
(SETU BANDHASANA)

- Lie on your back with your knees bent and feet parallel. The feet should be directly beneath the knees with equal pressure on the inner and outer edge of each foot.

- Bend your elbows as if you are holding a box right over your chest, and puff the chest up while pressing the elbows down.

- Lay your hands back down, press into the floor with your elbows and your feet and lift your hips. This is Bridge Pose.

- Keep your legs parallel, and if your knees are uncomfortable, try walking your feet 1–2 inches (3–5 centimeters) forward. If your back is uncomfortable, try walking your feet a little bit wider apart. You can keep your arms at your sides, or roll your shoulders underneath you, interlace your fingers, and press your arms down as you lift your torso and chest higher.

- Breathe 5 deep, slow breaths before slowly rolling down from the top vertebrae to the bottom.

- Rest by lying on your back with the soles of the feet together, one hand on your heart, and one hand on your belly. When you are finished, hug your knees to your chest and make slow circles to massage the lower back.

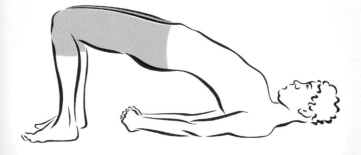

grounding

We are at our best when our life force has clear channels through which to flow and a path to follow. The origins of the path are the foundations, the secure roots from which we begin, expand, and ultimately flower. Think of any plant—the roots must be nourished with water and food before it can break through and receive the sun and air to complete its lifecycle. As you move through your practices, consider what seeds are taking root in your foundation and what has already provided you with inspiration and security. Practice Warrior II (see page 106) or the following variation on *Prithvi Mudra*.

PRITHVI MUDRA VARIATION
(EARTH MUDRA)

- Sit on the ground in a comfortable meditation position. Bring your thumb and ring finger together on each hand in *Prithvi Mudra* (see page 68).

- Sit tall and stretch your arms out by your sides with the fingers touching the floor.

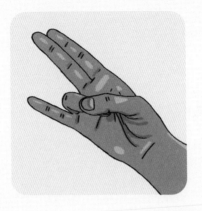

- Imagine your spine lifting skyward on the inhale and your energy lifting with it. On your exhale, stay lifted and imagine roots growing from every part of your body that is touching the floor. Feel the gentle tug as you connect more deeply to earth energy. Let it nourish and center you for 5 breaths.

- Maintaining the mudra, turn the hands to face up and place them with the arms extended on your legs. Hold for another 1–3 minutes.

connection

No matter what our spiritual beliefs may be, it is not too difficult to imagine that we share a common home, this planet Earth, and that we spring from a common source. To have a connection to something beyond ourselves is to experience belonging and support, and to diminish feelings of isolation. We see more clearly that we are essential, universal, and unique.

If we can stay in touch with our own divine essence, we have endless source energy at our fingertips with which we can shape the world into its most harmonious, peaceful, and vibrant manifestation.

OM
(AUM)

The mantra of Om is said to represent everything from the most infinitesimal aspect of creation to the most omnipotent. As with all yoga practice, this is not a religious mantra. It is an invocation, an honoring of the seed of creation, and represents our life journey, all that came before, and all that comes after.

Its full symbolism is displayed when written as...

**A (Ahhh): the beginning,
or energy of creation.**

**U (Ooohh): maintaining,
or energy of sustaining.**

**M (Mmmm): the deconstruction,
or energy of transformation.**

When we chant and contemplate "om," we are opening to a deeper sense of being. After all, we are human beings, not human doings.

CHANT OM

- Sit comfortably in *Sukhasana* (see page 16) with your hands relaxed naturally or in *Jnana Mudra* with the thumb and index finger touching. Close your eyes.

- Bring your third eye—the sixth chakra (see page 142), the space between your eyebrows—into your awareness. Take a few moments to focus on that point. You may even be able to visualize the color indigo or a shade of purple there.

- When you feel ready, begin to chant "Ommm..."

resources

There are so many glorious and informative books and articles that I feel have shaped and touched my teaching that it could be an endless list. However, the following are the most direct sources that made their way either into the pages or into the spirit of the book.

- *Pocketful of Miracles* by Joan Borysenko (Warner Books, 1994)

- *Mudras: Yoga in Your Hands* by Gertrud Hirschi (Red Wheel/Weiser, 2016)

- *Light on Yoga* by B. K. S. Iyengar (Schocken Books, 1979)

- *Yoga: The Path to Holistic Health* by B. K. S. Iyengar (Dorling Kindersley, 2014)

- *Healing Mudras: Yoga for Your Hands* by Sabrina Mesko (The Ballantine Publishing Group, 2000)

- *The Anatomy of the Spirit* by Caroline Myss (Three Rivers Press, 1996)

- *The Yoga Sutras of Patanjali* by Sri Swami Satchidananda (Integral Yoga Publications, 1999)

- *The Book of Chakras* by Ambika Wauters (Quarto Publishing, 2002)

- *Yoga Beyond Belief* by Ganga White (North Atlantic Books, 2007)

You can find out more about my yoga classes and reach me at **christineburkeyoga.com**, **liberationyoga. com**, and **@liberationyoga** on Instagram and Facebook.

CHAKRAS

Chakras are energy centers in the body that correspond to our physical, emotional, and mental balance. In Sanskrit, chakra means "wheel," signifying that our life force (prana) is spinning inside us like a wheel of light. Through yoga, we can open any chakras that are blocked and achieve a healthy state where all of our chakras are balanced. This diagram may give you a more tangible idea of how your practices will tap into your whole being in a powerful way.

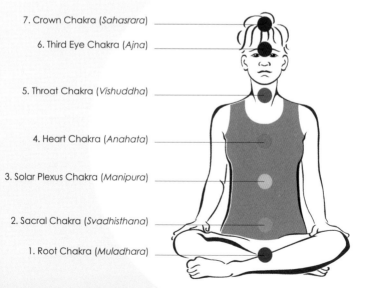

7. Crown Chakra (*Sahasrara*)

6. Third Eye Chakra (*Ajna*)

5. Throat Chakra (*Vishuddha*)

4. Heart Chakra (*Anahata*)

3. Solar Plexus Chakra (*Manipura*)

2. Sacral Chakra (*Svadhisthana*)

1. Root Chakra (*Muladhara*)

index of poses

INDEX OF POSES

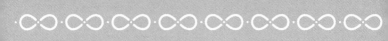